I0791556

**ISBN:** 9781673219159

# 7-Day Diet For Men

**Gail Johnson, M.S.**
**Ron Hill, Jr.**

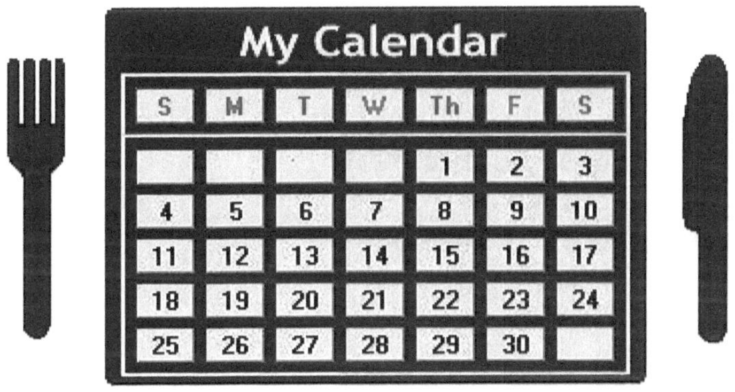


**NoPaperPress™**

**Note:** At publication, the off-the-shelf foods used in some of this book were widely available in most supermarkets. But food products come and go. So if there is a frozen entrée or soup selection in this diet that is out of stock, or that's been discontinued, or perhaps you don't like, or that you forgot to pick up while shopping, please substitute another food that has **approximately** the same caloric value and nutritional content. In this regard, many dieters have found the foods listed in the Appendices at the end of this book to be very helpful.

# CONTENTS

## When to Use the 7-Day Diet

If you're in weight maintenance mode but notice your weight creeping up. You want to stop the upward trend and lose a few kilos as well. Here's the perfect solution: Use the *7-Day Diet* to quickly lose unwanted weight!

Maybe you've let your weight get out of control and decide to go on a diet. It doesn't matter what diet, or how much weight you want to lose. Your first move should be to go on the 7-*Day Diet* lose a few pounds and get on the right track. After the 7-day diet does its job you can switch to a longer-term diet. My suggestion would be the *30-Day Quick Diet – For Men* also published by NoPaperPress.

Additionally, before you begin any weight loss program you should know your current health status. Assessing your cardio (aerobic) capacity, your percent body-fat, and even how appropriate your nutritional practices are, will help you establish what you should emphasize in a weight control program and help you set goals. You also need to make sure your health will allow you to lower your caloric intake and increase your physical activity. A medical checkup is in order which may be as simple as a visit to a physician who is familiar with your medical history, or it may be a thorough physical exam. The physician conducting the medical exam should be made aware of and should approve the specific weight loss diet you're planning.

## What's in this eBook?

**This eBook actually contains two 7-day diets: a 1,500 Calorie diet, and for even faster weight loss a 1,200 Calorie diet.** Both diets have a meal plan (menu) for each and every day. And every day features a "Recipe and Diet Tip of the Day."

## Which Calorie Level is for You?

**1,200 Calorie Diet:** Smaller men, older men and inactive men should select the 1,200 Calorie diet.
**1,500 Calorie Diet:** Larger men, younger men and active men should choose the 1,500 Calorie diet.

## How Much Weight Will You Lose?

Weight loss occurs when your food energy intake is less than the total energy you expend. This difference in calories is referred to as your calorie deficit. How much weight you lose depends on the magnitude of your calorie deficit. Physiologists have long known that to lose one pound requires a deficit of approximately 3,500 Calories. Therefore, if a person's total calorie deficit over time is known, their weight loss over time can be calculated.

**On the 7-Day Diet, most men lose 4 to 5 pounds** – depending on whether the 1,200 or 1,500 Calorie diet is selected. Smaller men, older men and less active men will lose a bit less and larger men, younger men and more active men somewhat more.  Exactly how much weight you will lose depends on how much you weigh, your age and your activity level.  For the full story see *Weight Control - U.S. Edition* by Vincent Antonetti, Ph.D.

## How to Use This eBook

First, depending on  your size, your age and how active you are, choose the diet calorie level that's right for you, either 1200 or 1,500 Calories per day.
- **1200-Calorie Diet Daily Menus go to page 9.**
- **1500-Calorie Diet Daily Menus go to page 17.**
Next, study the meal plan for the calorie level you have selected and then scan the appropriate Food Shopping List. Finally, using the food shopping list prepare a list of the foods you don't have on hand – that you will need to buy.
- **1200 and 1500-Calorie Shopping Tips** go to page 33.

# 1200 Calorie Daily Menus

# Day 1 – 1200 Calorie Meal Plan

| BREAKFAST | Calories | Totals |
|---|---|---|
| Cantaloupe (½ medium) | 50 | |
| Wheaties (¾ cup) + ½ cup skim milk + ½ banana | 190 | |
| Coffee (Notes page 39) | 10 | 250 Cal |
| | | |
| **SNACK** | | |
| Coffee or tea | 10 | 10 Cal |
| **LUNCH** | | |
| Soup (Appendix C - page 41) | 140 | |
| Turkey breast (1 oz) on 1 slice rye bread) | 115 | |
| Pickle spear | 0 | |
| Lettuce & tomato slices | 20 | |
| Hot or iced tea | 10 | 285 Cal |
| | | |
| **SNACK** | | |
| Coffee or tea | 10 | 10 Cal |
| **DINNER** | | |
| Baked salmon with salsa (Day 1 Recipe - page 25) | 215 | |
| Summer squash, zucchini and tomatoes | 60 | |
| Brown rice (½ cup) | 100 | |
| Large tossed green salad w 1½ Tbsp low-cal dressing* | 70 | |
| Fresh fruit in season (apple, peach, etc) | 70 | |
| Water | 0 | 515 Cal |
| | | |
| * See **Dinner Guidelines** - page 37 | | |
| **SNACK** | | |
| Fiber One Chocolate Fudge Brownie | 90 | |
| Skim milk (4 oz) | 45 | 135 Cal |
| | | |
| | | 1205 Cal |

# Day 2 – 1200 Calorie Meal Plan

| BREAKFAST | Calories | Totals |
|---|---|---|
| Orange juice (½ cup) | 50 | |
| Soft-boiled egg | 80 | |
| Whole-grain toast (1 slice) (See **Notes**) | 65 | |
| Coffee | 10 | 205 Cal |
| | | |
| **SNACK** | | |
| Coffee or tea | 10 | 10 Cal |
| **LUNCH** | | |
| Salad (3 oz tuna, 1 tsp Evoo, onions & celery) | 175 | |
| Lettuce & tomato wedges | 20 | |
| Rye bread ( 1 slice) | 65 | |
| Fresh fruit in season (apple, peach, etc) | 70 | |
| Coffee or tea | 10 | 340 Cal |
| | | |
| **SNACK** | | |
| Yogurt (6 oz, nonfat, any flavor)* | 90 | |
| Coffee or tea | 10 | 100 Cal |
| | | |
| **DINNER** | | |
| Veggie burger – (1 patty) (Day 2 Recipe - page 26) | 100 | |
| Low-fat cheddar cheese (1 thin slice) | 50 | |
| Seeded hamburger roll | 140 | |
| Large tossed green salad w 1½ Tbsp low-cal dressing | 70 | |
| Fresh fruit in season (apple, plum, etc) | 70 | |
| Water with lemon section | 15 | 445 Cal |
| | | |
| **SNACK** | | |
| Fiber One Chocolate Fudge Brownie | 90 | |
| Coffee or tea | 10 | 100 Cal |
| | | |
| * For example, Dannon Lite & Fit.  (Buy 32 oz use 6 oz.) | | **1200 Cal** |

# Day 3 – 1200 Calorie Meal Plan

| BREAKFAST | Calories | Totals |
|---|---|---|
| Orange juice (½ cup) | 50 | |
| Wild blueberry pancakes (Day 3 Recipe - page 27) | 190 | |
| Light syrup (2 Tbsp) | 60 | |
| Coffee | 10 | 310 Cal |
| | | |
| **SNACK** | | |
| Coffee or tea | 10 | 10 Cal |
| | | |
| **LUNCH** | | |
| Peanut butter (2 Tbsp) on 2 slices bread | 330 | |
| Skim milk (6 oz) | 70 | |
| Small bunch of grapes | 50 | 450 Cal |
| | | |
| **SNACK** | | |
| Coffee or tea | 10 | 10 Cal |
| | | |
| **DINNER** | | |
| Broiled pork chop (½" thick & trimmed of all fat) | 260 | |
| Green peas (½ cup) | 55 | |
| Large tossed green salad w 1½ Tbsp low-cal dressing | 70 | |
| Water with lemon section | 15 | 400 Cal |
| | | |
| **SNACK** | | |
| Coffee or tea | 10 | 10 Cal |
| | | |
| | | 1190 Cal |

# Day 4 – 1200 Calorie Meal Plan

| BREAKFAST | Calories | Totals |
|---|---|---|
| Fresh sliced orange | 75 | |
| Cheerios (1 cup) + ½ cup skim milk + 15 raisins* | 190 | |
| Coffee | 10 | 275 Cal |
| | | |
| **SNACK** | | |
| Fresh fruit in season (apple, plum, etc) | 70 | |
| Coffee or tea | 10 | 80 Cal |
| | | |
| **LUNCH** | | |
| Cottage cheese (1 cup low fat) | 180 | |
| Large tossed salad with 1½ Tbsp low-cal dressing | 70 | |
| Small whole-grain roll | 80 | |
| Hot or iced tea | 10 | 340 Cal |
| | | |
| **SNACK** | | |
| Handful unsalted mixed nuts | 100 | 100 Cal |
| | | |
| **DINNER** | | |
| Grilled chicken sausage (2 links - 2½ oz per link) | 180 | |
| Artichoke-bean salad (Day 4 Recipe - page 28) | 190 | |
| Green beans - steamed | 25 | |
| Water | 0 | 395 Cal |
| | | |
| **SNACK** | | |
| Coffee or tea | 10 | 10 Cal |
| | | |
| * You may substitute 2 blueberries per raisin. | | 1200 Cal |

# Day 5 – 1200 Calorie Meal Plan

| BREAKFAST | Calories | Totals |
|---|---|---|
| Cantaloupe (½ medium) | 50 | |
| Scrambled egg (Notes - page 39) | 80 | |
| Whole-grain toast (1 slice) | 65 | |
| Coffee | 10 | 205 Cal |
| | | |
| **SNACK** | | |
| Yogurt (6 oz, nonfat, any flavor) | 90 | |
| Coffee or tea | 10 | 100 Cal |
| | | |
| **LUNCH** | | |
| Subway 6" (Ham, Cheese +veggies)* | 260 | |
| Hot or iced tea | 10 | 270 Cal |
| | | |
| **SNACK** | | |
| Coffee or tea | 10 | 10 Cal |
| | | |
| **DINNER** | | |
| Frozen Entree (Day 5 Recipe - page 29) | 300 | |
| Large tossed salad w 1½ Tbsp low-cal dressing | 70 | |
| Fresh fruit in season (peach, plum, etc) | 70 | |
| Water with lemon section | 15 | 455 Cal |
| | | |
| **SNACK** | | |
| Two small cookies | 150 | |
| Coffee or tea | 10 | 160 Cal |
| | | |
| | | 1200 Cal |

# Day 6 – 1200 Calorie Meal Plan

| BREAKFAST | Calories | Totals |
|---|---|---|
| Orange juice (½ cup) | 50 | |
| Fried egg | 80 | |
| Whole-grain toast (1 slice) | 65 | |
| Coffee | 10 | 205 Cal |
| | | |
| **SNACK** | | |
| Yogurt (6 oz, nonfat, any flavor) | 90 | |
| Coffee or tea | 10 | 100 Cal |
| | | |
| **LUNCH** | | |
| Grilled Swiss cheese sandwich (2 oz low-fat cheese) | 310 | |
| Pickle spear | 0 | |
| Hot or iced tea | 10 | 320 Cal |
| | | |
| **SNACK** | | |
| Fresh fruit in season (apple, plum, etc) | 70 | |
| Coffee or tea | 10 | 80 Cal |
| | | |
| **DINNER** | | |
| Baked Herb-Crusted Cod (Day 6 Recipe - page 31) | 230 | |
| Asparagus (7 spears cooked & drained) | 20 | |
| Large tossed green salad w 1½ Tbsp low-cal dressing | 70 | |
| Water with lemon section | 15 | 335 Cal |
| | | |
| **SNACK** | | |
| Dark chocolate (1 oz) | 150 | |
| Coffee or tea | 10 | 160 Cal |
| | | |
| | | 1200 Cal |

# Day 7 – 1200 Calorie Meal Plan

| BREAKFAST | Calories | Totals |
|---|---|---|
| Orange juice (½ cup) | 50 | |
| Shredded Wheat (1 cup) + ½ cup milk + ½ banana | 260 | |
| Coffee | 10 | 320 Cal |
| | | |
| **SNACK** | | |
| Coffee or tea | 10 | 10 Cal |
| | | |
| **LUNCH** | | |
| Turkey frank (2 oz) with mustard & relish | 150 | |
| Hot dog bun | 130 | |
| Gelatin dessert (unsweetened) | 10 | |
| Hot or iced tea | 10 | 300 Cal |
| | | |
| **SNACK** | | |
| Yogurt (6 oz, nonfat, any flavor) | 90 | |
| Coffee or tea | 10 | 100 Cal |
| | | |
| **DINNER** | | |
| Pasta with Marinara sauce (Day 7 Recipe - page 32) | 225 | |
| Large tossed green salad with 1½ Tbsp low-cal | 70 | |
| Fresh fruit in season (pear, plum, etc) | 70 | |
| Italian or French bread (1 slice) | 80 | |
| Water with lemon section | 15 | 460 Cal |
| | | |
| **SNACK** | | |
| Coffee or tea | 10 | 10 Cal |
| | | |
| | | 1200 Cal |

# 1500 Calorie Daily Menus

# Day 1– 1,500 Calorie Meal Plan

| BREAKFAST | Calories | Totals |
|---|---|---|
| Cantaloupe (½ medium) | 50 | |
| Wheaties (¾ cup) + ½ cup skim milk + ½ banana | 190 | |
| Whole-grain toast (1 slice) (Notes - page 39) | 65 | |
| Coffee (Notes) | 10 | 315 Cal |
| | | |
| SNACK | | |
| Fresh fruit in season ( peach, plum, etc) | 70 | 70 Cal |
| | | |
| LUNCH | | |
| Soup (Appendix C - page 41) | 140 | |
| Turkey breast (1 oz) on 1 slice rye bread | 115 | |
| Lettuce & tomato slices | 20 | |
| Hot or iced tea | 10 | 285 Cal |
| | | |
| SNACK | | |
| Two small cookies | 160 | |
| Skim milk (4 oz) | 45 | 205 Cal |
| | | |
| DINNER | | |
| Baked salmon with salsa (Day 1 Recipe - page 25) | 215 | |
| Summer squash, zucchini and tomatoes | 60 | |
| Brown rice (½ cup) | 100 | |
| Large tossed green salad w 1½ Tbsp low-cal dressing* | 70 | |
| Fresh fruit in season (apple, peach, etc) | 70 | |
| Water | 0 | 515 Cal |
| | | |
| * See **Dinner Guidelines** - page 37 | | |
| Hot or iced tea | 10 | 270 Cal |
| Handful unsalted mixed nuts | 100 | |
| Coffee or tea | 10 | 110 Cal |
| | | |
| | | 1500 Cal |

# Day 2 – 1,500 Calorie Meal Plan

| BREAKFAST | Calories | Totals |
|---|---|---|
| Orange juice (½ cup) | 50 | |
| Soft-boiled egg | 80 | |
| Whole-grain toast (2 slices) (Notes - page 39) | 130 | |
| Coffee | 10 | 270 Cal |
| | | |
| **SNACK** | | |
| Yogurt (6 oz, nonfat, any flavor)* | 90 | |
| Coffee or tea | 10 | 100 Cal |
| **LUNCH** | | |
| Salad (3 oz tuna, 1 tsp Evoo, onions & celery) | 175 | |
| Lettuce & tomato wedges + rye bread ( 1 slice) | 85 | |
| Fresh fruit in season (apple, peach, etc) | 70 | |
| Lettuce & tomato wedges + rye bread ( 1 slice) | 10 | |
| Coffee or tea | 10 | 350 Cal |
| | | |
| **SNACK** | | |
| Handful unsalted mixed nuts | 100 | |
| Coffee or tea | 10 | 110 Cal |
| **DINNER** | | |
| Veggie burger – (1 patty) (Day 2 Recipe - page 26) | 100 | |
| Low-fat cheddar cheese (1 thin slice) | 50 | |
| Seeded hamburger roll | 140 | |
| Large tossed green salad w 1½ Tbsp low-cal dressing | 70 | |
| Beets (3 small) | 45 | |
| Fresh fruit in season (apple, plum, etc) | 70 | |
| Hot or iced tea | 10 | 485 Cal |
| | | |
| **SNACK** | | |
| Graham crackers (4 squares) | 120 | |
| Skim milk (6 oz) | 70 | 190 Cal |
| | | |
| * Such as Dannon Lite & Fit.  (Buy 32 oz use 6 oz.) | | 1505 Cal |

# Day 3 – 1,500 Calorie Meal Plan

| BREAKFAST | Calories | Totals |
|---|---|---|
| Cantaloupe (½ medium) | 50 | |
| Wild blueberry pancakes (**Day 3 Recipe -** page 27) | 190 | |
| Turkey bacon (2 slices) (Notes) | 70 | |
| Light syrup (1 Tbsp) | 30 | |
| Coffee | 10 | 365 Cal |
| | | |
| **SNACK** | | |
| Yogurt (6 oz, nonfat, any flavor) | 90 | |
| Coffee or tea | 10 | 100 Cal |
| | | |
| **LUNCH** | | |
| Peanut butter (2 Tbsp) on 2 slices bread | 330 | |
| Skim milk (6 oz) | 70 | |
| Fresh fruit in season (peach, pear, etc) | 70 | 470 Cal |
| | | |
| **SNACK** | | |
| Carrot sticks + ¼ cup low-fat cottage cheese & chives | 60 | 60 Cal |
| | | |
| **DINNER** | | |
| Broiled pork chop (about ½" thick & trimmed of fat) | 260 | |
| Green peas (½ cup) | 55 | |
| Tomato & cucumber salad w 1½Tbsp low-cal dressing | 70 | |
| Water | 0 | 385 Cal |
| | | |
| **SNACK** | | |
| Graham crackers (4 squares) | 120 | |
| Coffee or tea | 10 | 130 Cal |
| | | |
| | | 1510 Cal |

# Day 4 – 1,500 Calorie Meal Plan

| BREAKFAST | Calories | Totals |
|---|---|---|
| Fresh sliced orange | 75 | |
| Cheerios (1 cup) + ½ cup skim milk + 15 raisins* | 190 | |
| Whole-grain toast (1 slice) | 65 | |
| Coffee | 10 | 340 Cal |
| | | |
| **SNACK** | | |
| Fresh fruit in season (pear, plum, etc) | 70 | |
| Coffee or tea | 10 | 80 Cal |
| | | |
| **LUNCH** | | |
| Cottage cheese (1 cup low fat) | 180 | |
| Large tossed salad with 1½ Tbsp low-cal dressing | 70 | |
| Small whole-grain roll | 80 | |
| Hot or iced tea | 10 | 340 Cal |
| | | |
| **SNACK** | | |
| Handful unsalted mixed nuts | 100 | |
| Coffee or tea | 10 | 110 Cal |
| | | |
| **DINNER** | | |
| Grilled chicken sausage (2 links - 2½ oz per link) | 180 | |
| Artichoke-bean salad (Day 4 Recipe - page 28) | 190 | |
| Green beans - steamed | 25 | |
| Whole-grain bread (1 slice) | 65 | |
| Water with lemon section | 15 | 475 Cal |
| | | |
| **SNACK** | | |
| Two small cookies | 150 | |
| Coffee or tea | 10 | 160 Cal |
| | | |
| * You may substitute 2 blueberries per raisin. | | 1505 Cal |

# Day 5 – 1,500 Calorie Meal Plan

| BREAKFAST | Calories | Totals |
|---|---|---|
| Grapefruit (½) | 75 | |
| Scrambled egg (**Notes -** page 39) | 80 | |
| Turkey bacon (2 slices) | 70 | |
| Whole-grain toast (1 slice) | 65 | |
| Coffee | 10 | 300 Cal |
| | | |
| **SNACK** | | |
| Yogurt (6 oz, nonfat, any flavor) | 90 | |
| Coffee or tea | 10 | 100 Cal |
| | | |
| **LUNCH** | | |
| Chicken, Broccoli & Cheese* | 270 | |
| Gelatin dessert (unsweetened) | 10 | |
| Hot or iced tea | 10 | 290 Cal |
| | | |
| * Hot Pockets (wrap) | | |
| **SNACK** | | |
| Handful unsalted mixed nuts | 100 | |
| Coffee or tea | 10 | 110 Cal |
| | | |
| **DINNER** | | |
| Frozen Entree (**Day 5 Recipe -** page 29) | 300 | |
| Large tossed salad with 1½ Tbsp low-cal dressing | 70 | |
| Whole-grain bread (1 slice) | 65 | |
| Fresh fruit in season (apple, peach, etc) | 70 | |
| Water with lemon section | 15 | 520 Cal |
| | | |
| **SNACK** | | |
| Two small cookies | 160 | |
| Coffee or tea | 10 | 170 Cal |
| | | |
| | | 1490 Cal |

# Day 6 – 1,500 Calorie Meal Plan

| BREAKFAST | Calories | Totals |
|---|---|---|
| Grapefruit (½) | 75 | |
| Wheaties (¾ cup) + ½ cup skim milk + banana | 240 | |
| Whole-grain toast (1 slice) | 65 | |
| Coffee | 10 | 390 Cal |
| | | |
| **SNACK** | | |
| Fresh fruit in season (apple, plum, etc) | 70 | |
| Coffee or tea | 10 | 80 Cal |
| | | |
| **LUNCH** | | |
| Grilled Swiss cheese sandwich (2 oz low-fat cheese) | 310 | |
| Gelatin dessert (unsweetened) | 10 | |
| Pickle spear | 0 | |
| Hot or iced tea | 10 | 330 Cal |
| | | |
| **SNACK** | | |
| Handful unsalted mixed nuts | 100 | |
| Coffee or tea | 10 | 110 Cal |
| | | |
| **DINNER** | | |
| Baked Herb-Crusted Cod *(Day 6 Recipe - page 31) | 230 | |
| Asparagus (7 spears cooked & drained) | 20 | |
| Large tossed green salad w 1½ Tbsp low-cal dressing | 70 | |
| Yogurt (6 oz nonfat, any flavor) | 90 | |
| Water with lemon section | 15 | 425 Cal |
| | | |
| **SNACK** | | |
| Dark chocolate (1 oz) | 150 | |
| Coffee or tea | 10 | 160 Cal |
| | | |
| | | 1495 Cal |

# Day 7 – 1,500 Calorie Meal Plan

| BREAKFAST | Calories | Totals |
|---|---|---|
| Orange juice (½ cup) | 50 | |
| Shredded Wheat (1 cup) + ½ cup milk + ½ banana | 260 | |
| Coffee | 10 | 320 Cal |
| | | |
| **SNACK** | | |
| Handful unsalted mixed nuts | 100 | |
| Coffee or tea | 10 | 110 Cal |
| | | |
| **LUNCH** | | |
| Turkey frank (2 oz) with mustard & relish | 150 | |
| Hot dog bun | 130 | |
| Diet soda or water | 0 | 280 Cal |
| | | |
| **SNACK** | | |
| Yogurt (6 oz, nonfat, any flavor) | 90 | |
| Coffee or tea | 10 | 100 Cal |
| | | |
| **DINNER** | | |
| Pasta with Marinara sauce (Day 7 Recipe - page 32) | 225 | |
| Large tossed green salad w 1½ Tbsp low-cal dressing | 70 | |
| Fresh fruit in season (apple, plum, etc) | 70 | |
| Italian or French bread (1 slice) | 80 | |
| Glass of red wine (4 oz) | 100 | |
| Water with lemon section | 15 | 560 Cal |
| | | |
| **SNACK** | | |
| Graham crackers (4 squares) | 120 | |
| Coffee or tea | 10 | 130 Cal |
| | | |
| | | 1500 Cal |

# Recipes & Diet Tips

# Day 1 Recipe

## Baked Salmon with Salsa

This is a simple, straight-forward recipe.  The advantage of a simple recipe is that there are no hidden calories.

>    4 - 5 oz salmon fillets

>    6 - Tbsp bottled tomato-pepper salsa

Brown salmon fillets in non-stick pan and place in baking dish.  Put fillets in an oven preheated to 350 ºF for about 10 minutes.  Plate the salmon.  Stir prepared tomato-pepper salsa and spoon it over the salmon.

<u>Serves 4</u>.  One salmon fillet is about 215 Calories.

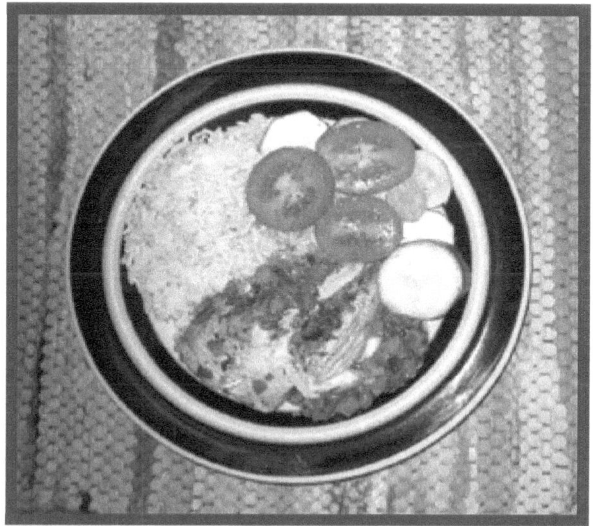

<u>Diet Tip of the Day:</u> **Have soup more often.**  Most <u>non-cream-based</u> soups are filling and low-calorie.

<h1 align="center">Day 2 Recipe</h1>

## Veggie Burger

Vegetable-based burgers can be purchased at your local supermarket. The patty of a veggie burger can be made from vegetables, soy, nuts, mushrooms, textured vegetable protein, dairy, or a combination of these foods.

Two popular veggie burgers are the Boca Burger and Gardenburger. The Boca Burger is made chiefly from soy protein and wheat gluten. (Boca Burger patties are 2.5 oz each and range from 60 to 90 Calories.) The original Gardenburger is made from mushrooms, onions, brown rice, rolled oats, cheese, and spices. (Gardenburger patties are 2.5 oz each and about 100 Calories.)

To prepare, follow package directions. The version shown below has an added slice of low-fat cheddar cheese. The lettuce, tomato and ketchup shown actually add very few extra calories.

The veggie burger patty plus low-fat cheese amounts to approximately 150 Calories. Add a seeded roll and the total rises to 290 Calories.

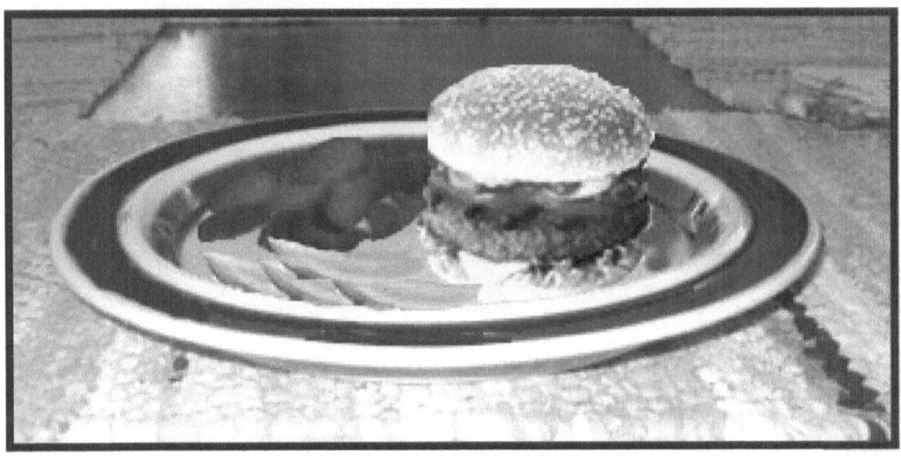

<u>**Diet Tip of the Day:**</u> **Drink lots of water** – about 8 glasses per day. Add a slice of lemon to make it more interesting. Often, when you think you're hungry, you are just thirsty. So, next time you head for a snack, drink some water first and see if that does it for you.

# Day 3 Recipe

## Wild Blueberry Pancakes

This recipe makes a relatively low calorie, wholesome batch of delicious wild blueberry-whole wheat-buttermilk pancakes.

- 1 - cup whole-wheat flour
- 1 - cup buttermilk
- 1 - egg
- 1 - Tbsp vegetable oil
- 1 - tsp baking powder
- ½ - tsp baking soda

Stir ingredients until blended.  Add ¾ cup blueberries and gently stir.  Using medium heat, preheat a non-stick skillet coated with cooking spray.  Pour slightly less than ¼ cup of batter onto skillet per pancake.  Cook slowly until bubbles break on surface of pancake.  Turn and cook until other side is lightly browned.  Makes 8 pancakes.

**Serves 4**.  Each pancake is about 95 Calories.  Pictured below are wild-blueberry pancakes with two slices of turkey bacon.

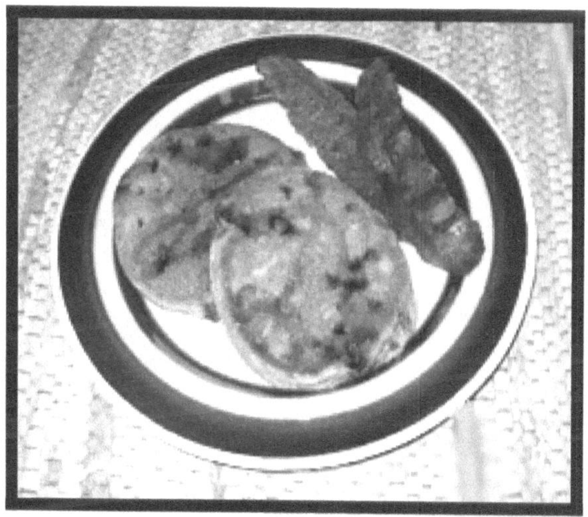

**Diet Tip of the Day:**  A peanut butter sandwich on whole wheat bread with a glass of skim milk and an apple makes a nutritious, reasonably low-calorie lunch.

# Day 4 Recipe

## Artichoke-Bean Salad

    1 - can (19 oz) white kidney beans
    10 - artichoke hearts, quartered
    ⅓ - cup chopped oregano
    ⅓ - cup chopped parsley
    3 - cloves garlic, chopped
    1 - lemon, juiced

Combine ingredients in medium-size bowl.  Stir in ¼ cup Evoo.  Salt and black pepper to taste.

**Serves 6**.  Approximately 190 Calories per serving.  Pictured on the plate below are two grilled chicken sausage links with salsa, steamed green beans and the artichoke-bean salad.  Incidentally, the artichoke-bean combination over mixed salad greens served with a whole-grain bread makes a delicious, nutritious and reasonable low-calorie main course.

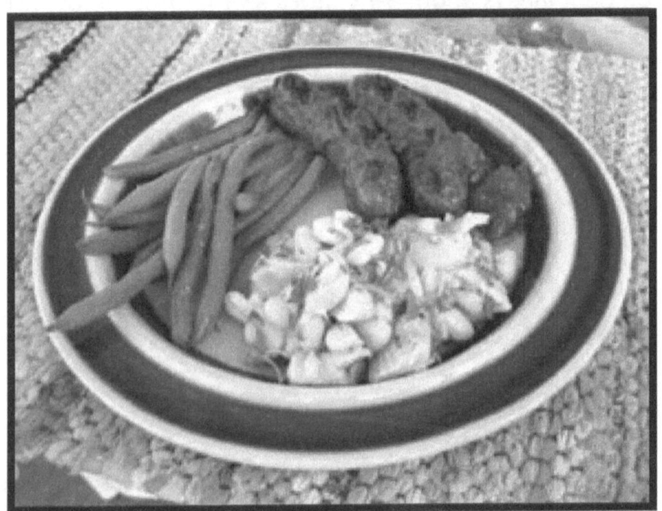

**Diet Tip of the Day:**  Have a small meal before you go to a party.  A hardboiled egg, an apple, and a thirst quencher (like water, tea, seltzer, or diet soda) will take the edge off your appetite and make it easier to resist the high-calorie goodies.

# Day 5 Recipe

No recipe today.  The **frozen dinner** for Day 5, for both the 1,200 and 1500-Calorie diets, is any one of the following:

| Poultry | Sweet Sesame Chicken | Healthy Choice | 300 |
|---|---|---|---|
| Poultry | Chicken Fettuccini | Smart Ones | 300 |
| Poultry | Spicy Chicken Strips & Fries | Smart Ones | 300 |
| Meat | Classic Meat Loaf | Healthy Choice | 300 |
| Seafood | Tortilla Crusted Fish | Lean Cuisine | 300 |
| Pasta | Garlic Sesame Noodles with Beef | Lean Cuisine | 300 |

In some instances, frozen may actually be better than fresh, because if you keep fresh fruit and vegetables in your fridge for a long time, they lose some of their nutritional value.  Whereas, frozen foods are usually processed and packaged within hours of being picked.  And the freezing process itself does not destroy nutrients.  So buying frozen and then defrosting when you want the fruit or vegetable can actually retain more nutrients.

According to the U.S. Department of Agriculture, food stored continuously at 0 °F is always safe to eat.  Freezing keeps food safe and preserves food for extended periods because it prevents the growth of microorganisms that cause food spoilage and illness.  **Please read the important Frozen-Food Safety Warning in Appendix E.**

Use an appliance thermometer to monitor your freezer's temperature.  If a refrigerator freezing compartment can't maintain 0° F or if the freezer door is opened frequently, use it for short-term food storage, and eat those foods as soon as possible for best quality.  Use a free-standing freezer set at 0° F or below for long-term storage of frozen foods.  Again, keep a thermometer in your freezing compartment or freezer to check the temperature.

Because freezing keeps food safe almost indefinitely, recommended freezer storage times are to preserve quality (taste, etc) of food, not the safety or nutritional value.  **The quality of frozen dinners or entrees in a freezer at 0 °F will be maintained for 3 to 4 months**.

If there is a power outage, or if your freezer fails, or if the freezer door is left ajar by mistake, the food may still be safe to use.  As long as a freezer with its door ajar continues to run, to cool, the foods should stay safe overnight.  If a repairman is on the way or it appears the power will be restored soon, just keep your freezer door closed.  A freezer full of food will usually keep about 2 days if the door is kept shut; a half-full freezer will last about a day.  The freezing compartment of a refrigerator may not keep foods frozen as long .  If the freezer is not full, group packages together to help maintain their low temperature.

During a power failure, you may want to put dry ice, a block or bags of ice in the freezer, or transfer foods to a friend's freezer until power returns.  Again, use an appliance thermometer to monitor the temperature.  To determine the safety of foods when the power goes on, check their condition and temperature.  If food is partly frozen, still has ice crystals, or is as cold as if it were in a refrigerator (40 °F), it is safe to refreeze or use.  It's not necessary to cook raw foods before refreezing.  **If in doubt discard the food.  And always discard frozen food whose temperature has exceeded 40 °F for more than two hours.**

<u>**Diet Tip of the Day:**</u>  **Buy a pedometer** and start walking.  For the average person 2,100 steps amounts to walking about one mile.  A Harvard study has shown that 8,000 to 10,000 step per day promotes weight loss.

# Day 6 Recipe

## Baked Herb-Crusted Cod

   4 - 4 to 5 ounce cod fish fillets
   2 - tablespoons (Tbsp) flour
   2 - Tbsp cornmeal
   2 - Tbsp minced fresh herbs
   2 - teaspoons (tsp) lemon juice

Sprinkle cod with lemon juice. Mix flour, cornmeal and herbs and dust the cod with the cornmeal- herb mixture.  Bake in oven at 375 °F for 10 minutes. Add salt and black pepper to taste.

**Serves 4**. One serving is about 230 Calories (for cod only).

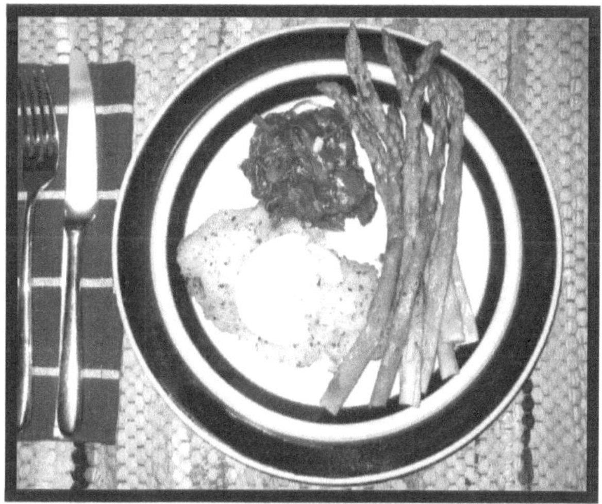

**Diet Tip of the Day:**  **Take a daily multi-vitamin/mineral supplement.**
This is important when you're on a diet – as a kind of insurance policy.

# Day 7 Recipe

## Pasta with Marinara Sauce

**Tomato sauce:** Sauté ½ small onion, chopped fine, in 1 tsp olive oil. Add two finely chopped garlic cloves, 1½ cups chopped plum tomatoes and ½ tsp chopped fresh oregano. Stir and cook about 5 minutes on a low flame. (Later add about ¼ cup of the pasta liquid to the sauce to thin it.)

    ½ pound <u>whole-wheat</u> pasta

    ¼ tsp salt

Bring 2 quarts of lightly salted water to a boil. Add pasta and stir occasionally (to keep pasta from sticking to the bottom of the pot). Keep water boiling and cook until pasta are "al dente." (Cooking time is approximately 9 minutes.) Drain pasta. (Remember to add some of the pasta liquid to the tomato sauce.) Pour the marinara sauce over the pasta and serve hot.

<u>Serves 4</u>. One serving is about 225 Calories.

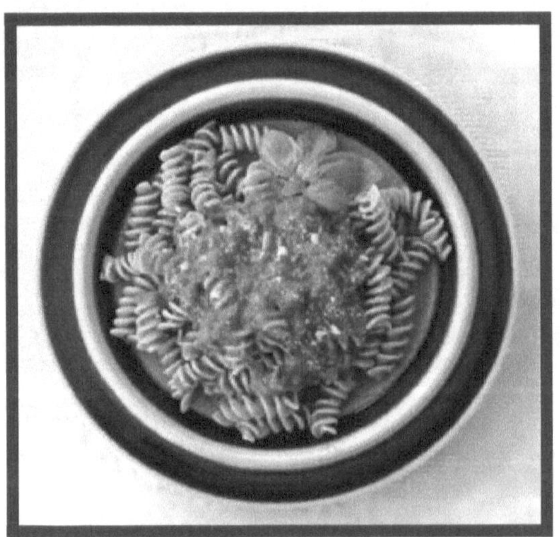

<u>**Diet Tip of the Day:**</u> **Beware of alcoholic beverages.** Beer has about 13 Calories per ounce, wine 25 Calories per ounce and whiskey 71 Calories per ounce.

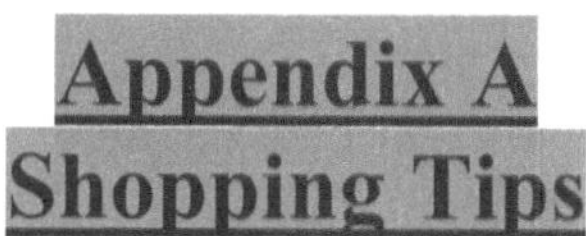

# Appendix A
# Shopping Tips

No cooking doesn't mean no preparation!  You will probably have to shop once a week.  The following should help you prepare your shopping list.

First, understand that the problem with basing a meal plan on name-brand food items, such as a particular Lean Cuisine frozen entree, is that the item might not be available where you shop, or it may have been discontinued. What to do? That's where Appendices C and D in this eBook come in handy. Appendix C lists 19 name-brand soups in microwaveable bowls. Appendix D lists more than 100 name-brand frozen meals with their calorie count. Using these lists you should be able to find a substitute for the soup or frozen entree you can't find - a substitute that is based on the same food type, e.g., chicken, fish, or meat, and has the same approximate calorie count.

## Exchanging Foods

If there is a food listed in the diet you don't like, or perhaps that you forgot to pick up while shopping, you probably can exchange or substitute another food in its place – a technique used by dieticians. Exchanging a food listed in a diet for another food with approximately equal caloric value and nutritional content is the foundation of a successful long-term diet.

Substitution possibilities are almost endless but have to be done carefully. The easiest substitutions are those within the same food group, such as exchanging one vegetable variety for another, or a glass of milk for a cup of yogurt. More sophisticated exchanges cross food groups, for instance replacing 3½ ounces of turkey with a tablespoon of peanut butter spread on a piece of whole wheat bread. Both foods are complete proteins and both contain about 175 Calories. Refer to a good online calorie table to find calorie values. With some understanding and experience, you will be able to substitute foods called for in this diet with equal calorie foods from the same food group.

Another alternative is the following Food Substitution List that suggests substitutions for a variety of food items that appear in the daily meal plans. For example, Day 5 of the diet calls for half a cantaloupe for breakfast. But suppose cantaloupe is not in season, or just doesn't look good, or maybe it's too expensive, or you can't find it at your grocery, from the Food Substitution List you find that you may exchange a ½ cup of orange juice for half cantaloupe – both are in the fruit category and both contain about 50 Calories.

**Light Syrup** - Use any light syrup (25 Calories per Tbsp)
**Big-Bowl Salad** - Exchange with unlimited steamed greens (spinach, etc)
**Cantaloupe** (½) - Use ½ cup Orange juice
**Cereal** - Exchange with any other whole-grain cereal
**Cottage Cheese** (1 cup) - Two 8 oz glasses skim milk
**Yogurt** - Select 6 ounces skim milk
**Eggs** – Use Egg Beaters
**Fresh fruit** - ¾ cup canned fruit (no sugar added)
**Frozen entrée** - Substitute frozen entrée with same calories.
**Grapefruit** (½) - Choose an orange (medium)
**Handful of Nuts** - Popcorn Mini Bag
**Kashi Chewy Granola Bar** - Quaker Chewy Dipps Granola Bar
**Kashi Go Lean Waffles** - Eggo Nutri-Grain Whole Wheat Frozen Waffles
**Hot Pockets Wraps** - Lean Pockets Wraps
**Morningstar Breakfast Sausage** - Any breakfast sausage with comparable calories
**String Cheese** - Laughing Cow light cheese (2 wedges)
**Popcorn** - Use handful of mixed nuts
**Raisin bread** - Plain whole-grain bread
**Skinny Cow Ice Cream Sandwich** - Skinny Cow Low Fat Fudge Bar
**Soup** - Choose any soup with same calorie count
**Whole-grain Bread** - Vary bread type (whole wheat, rye, etc)
**Wine** (4 oz) - Instead select grapes (1 cup)

## Guidelines for Healthy Eating

No single food can supply all the nutrients you need in the amounts you need. The most important factors in nutrition are variety, variety, variety! **Variety is the key to a nutritious diet.** As a means of setting strategies for food selection, the U.S. Department of Health and Human Services and the Department of Agriculture issue Dietary Guidelines every five years. The latest Dietary Guidelines describe a healthy diet as one that:
- Emphasizes fruits, vegetables, whole grains, and fat-free or low-fat milk products.
- Includes fish, poultry, lean meats, beans & nuts.
- Is low in saturated fats, trans fats, cholesterol, salt (sodium) and added sugars.

The guidelines encourage adults to consume a variety of nutrient-dense foods and beverages within their caloric needs. The afore mentioned U.S. government agencies recommends how much should be eaten from each of the basic food groups (i.e., from the fruit group, vegetable group, grains group, meat and beans group, milk group, and oils group) to meet your caloric goal – whether you are trying to lose weight or maintain weight. All this information and more can be found in my eBook *Eat Smart for Better Health - U.S. Edition* published by NoPaperPress.

Even though most adults can get all the vitamins and minerals they need by merely consuming a variety of nutritious foods (from the fruit group, the vegetable group, the grains group, the meat and beans group, the milk group, and the oils group), many physicians recommend a daily multi-vitamin/mineral supplement – just in case you don't eat the way you should.

Be aware that some micronutrients, such as the fat-soluble vitamin A, can be harmful if taken in large quantities. To be safe your multi-vitamin/mineral supplement should contain no more than 100 percent of the recommended dietary allowance (RDA) for each vitamin or mineral. Generally, you don't need the high doses in multi-vitamin/mineral supplements labeled "therapeutic" or "extra-strength." There may be medical reasons for taking larger amounts of a vitamin or mineral than the RDA provides, but check with your doctor first.

As you age, adequate protein intake and body protein reserves are more important than ever, especially during times of emotional and physical stress. Body proteins are constantly being made and used during your lifetime to maintain the functions of the cells and organs, and protein is needed to help to prevent muscle loss.  Good sources of protein-rich foods are meats, fish, eggs, dairy products, dried beans and peas, and soy products.  Vitamin $B_{12}$ can be a problem nutrient for older adults. Vitamin $B_{12}$ enables your body to manufacture healthy red-blood cells and assists in the transmission of electrical signals between nerve cells.  The acid in your stomach helps release vitamin $B_{12}$ from the protein in the food you eat.  This must occur before vitamin $B_{12}$ is absorbed in your intestines.  But as you age, the amount of stomach acid you produce decreases.  Less hydrochloric acid lessens the amount of vitamin $B_{12}$ separated from proteins in foods and can result in poor absorption of vitamin $B_{12}$.  Vitamin $B_{12}$ is found naturally in meat, fish, poultry, eggs and fortified cereals.  But recent  studies have revealed that up to 30 percent of adults aged 50 years and older may also have atrophic gastritis, an increased growth of intestinal bacteria, that renders them unable to normally absorb vitamin $B_{12}$ in food.  They are, however, able to absorb the synthetic vitamin $B_{12}$ added to fortified foods and dietary supplements.  As a result, fortified foods and vitamin supplements may be the best sources of vitamin $B_{12}$ for adults 50 years and older.

## What Makes for a Good Diet?

Every good weight-loss diet must have the following three characteristics: **First**, a good diet must provide you with an understanding of weight control as well as the knowledge you need to reduce your weight to the desired level. **Second**, a good diet must help you remain healthy while you are losing weight.  **Third**, a good diet must lead you to a healthier way of eating and exercising that will, in the long term, help you keep off the weight you have lost.

The weight-loss diet featured in this eBook is the so-called "balanced diet;" i.e., a diet that is not only low calorie and reasonably low in fat, but is also nutritionally balanced.  The *7-Day Diet for Men*, however, does not meet all the criteria set forth above.  While you will get some "dieting insight" and some idea of how much you can eat and still lose weight, you will not get a real understanding of weight control from this eBook.  That's not its purpose.  What you will get is a healthy diet – and a diet that if followed will promote weight loss.  Think of the *7-Day Diet* as a quick fix, a healthy start that will get you on the right track – but it's not the long-term answer.

**Long-term success** is about developing both an understanding and a plan that will result in healthier eating and physical activity habits.  The desire to lose weight and the discipline to start and stay on a weight-control program are crucial.  But along with desire and discipline, it is our belief that **only an in-depth understanding of weight control, nutrition and exercise will lead to**

**long-term success**.  For a through understanding and the guidance you need to succeed in the long term I recommend you read, *Weight Control – U.S. Edition* by Vincent W. Antonetti, Ph.D., an eBook also published by NoPaperPress.

## Breakfast Guidelines

You've heard it before.  It's important to start the day right and eat breakfast.  **So try to allow time for breakfast before you rush off to work.**  If need be do some preliminary preparation the night before such as setting up your coffee maker, deciding on and measuring the amount of cereal you will be eating, etc.  Many busy people prepare breakfast at home and bring it to work in a plastic container. Do what you need to do – but don't skip breakfast!

In the *7-Day Diet,* you may substitute wholesome **whole-grain cereal** for any specified cereal.  For example, if you're not crazy about having Shredded Wheat for breakfast on Day 6, substitute Wheat Chex or Cheerios, etc.  And if you don't like the fried egg called for on Day 5, have a hard-boiled egg or make a scrambled egg instead.  Maybe the cantaloupe called for in the meal plan is not in season.  No problem.  Just replace the cantaloupe with a half cup of orange juice.  Find a more complete list of food substitutions and exchanges page 34.

## Lunch Guidelines

On most days of the *7-Day Diet for Men,* lunch will call for either soup or a sandwich.  Feel free to substitute a soup you favor in place of those indicated – provided the basic type of soup and calorie counts are similar to those specified in the *7-Day Diet for Men.*  For example, Day 1 calls for a cup of Lentil Soup (140 Calories), but if you prefer, you may substitute a cup of Navy Bean Soup – which is in the same food group as lentil soup and contains approximately the same calorie count.

**Warm Weather Substitutions:** On warm and especially very hot days, you may want to substitute a sandwich, a tuna or salmon salad for the soup of the day.

## Dinner Guidelines

On the *7-Day Diet for Men*, one of the dinner mainstays is a "Tossed Green Salad." Prepare your "Tossed Green Salad" in a bowl with a volume of at least 16 ounces, or 2 cups.  First add about 1 cup of either green leaf lettuce, Romaine lettuce or a mesclun mix.  Then add, as desired, half cup of green veggies such as broccoli, celery, cucumber, peppers, spinach, or watercress. This vegetable combination will, on average, total about 35 Calories.  You will be eating a "Tossed Green Salad" just about every day at dinnertime.

Remember that variety is the key to a nutritious diet.  So be sure to vary the ingredients of the salad.

Top your "Tossed Green Salad" with 2 tablespoons of any light salad dressing available at your local supermarket that contains no more than 20 to 25 Calories per tablespoon.  Some of my favorite light salad dressings are:
   - **Ken's Steakhouse Fat Free Raspberry Pecan**
   - **Kraft Light Done Right House Italian**
   - **Wishbone Just 2 Good Honey Dijon**
   - **Newman's Lighten Up! Balsamic Vinaigrette**

Your "Tossed Green Salad" with salad dressing will cost you roughly 70 Calories but will be packed with lots of health-giving vitamins, minerals and fiber.

## Snack Guidelines

On some of the menus in the *7-Day Diet for Men* feature a morning snack, an afternoon snack and an evening snack.  The main snacks are:

**Yogurt:**  I recommend Dannon Light at 90 Calories per container (at this writing).  Select any flavor.  There are other brands you may prefer but whatever you buy be certain you eat no more than 90 Calories worth of yogurt for your snack.

**Fresh Fruit in season:** Choose an apple, pear, peach, plum, watermelon (1 cup), etc.  You will be eating fruit every day.  So vary the fruit that you select to get good array of micronutrients.

**Handful of Unsalted Mixed Nuts:** Nuts and seeds are loaded with protein and fiber.  This eBook uses a "handful" as a convenient descriptor rather than something like "16 almonds = 100 Calories," but be aware that although nuts are a healthy food, nuts are also a high-calorie food. Buy mixed nuts to get a range of micronutrients.  And please no salt.

**Skinny Cow Ice Cream Sandwich:** This is a relatively low-calorie, low fat, yummy dairy-sweet snack.

**Kashi TLC Chewy Granola Bar:** A sweet treat packed with whole grains, nuts and seeds. The bar comes in four flavors – with each containing about 140 Calories.

**Popcorn:** Popcorn is a tasty, nutritious high-fiber, filling snack.  A Popcorn Mini Bag, such as Orville Redenbacher's Smart Pop is convenient and contains 110 Calories.  But for the best popcorn I suggest you purchase a hot-air popper which uses popping corn, a type of corn that bursts from the kernel and puffs up when heated.  A hot-air popper will make a large batch of popcorn in a few minutes.  For a snack, eat only 5 or 6 cups of the popcorn and store the remainder for another day.  At this writing, you can buy a hot-air popper for approximately $25.00.

## About Bread

First understand that bread, more specifically whole-grain breads, are good sources of complex carbohydrates and dietary fiber, as well as several B vitamins (thiamin, riboflavin, niacin, and folate), vitamin E, and minerals (iron, magnesium and selenium).

In recent years, however, sliced bread loaves have gotten larger, as have the bread slices inside these loaves. Just a few years ago the standard slice of bread contained about 70 Calories – now most are 100 plus Calories.

**The *7-Day Diet* requires whole-grain bread at 70 Calories per slice.** Quite a few bakers sell thin sliced or "light" sliced bread. The difficult part is finding a whole grain thin sliced or "light" bread (with about 70 Calories per slice). Whatever the brand, make sure the first word in the Ingredients list is "whole." "Pepperidge Farm Small Slice 100% Whole Wheat" is a good choice. It's whole grain, has 70 Calories per slice and it tastes good too.

## Important Notes

**1)** If desired, skim milk and a sugar substitute may be added to coffee or tea. Coffee or tea may be regular or decaf. And soy or almond milk may be used instead of cow's milk.

**2)** Fried eggs, scrambled eggs, or an omelet should be cooked in a pan coated with a non-stick cooking spray.

**3)** On bread, corn on the cob and baked potatoes, if desired, you may use a zero-calorie butter substitute spray. Do not use butter!

**4)** Cereals should be whole grain and preferably without added sugar. At the top of the list are Old-fashioned Oat Meal, Wheatena and Shredded Wheat. Among other reasonably healthy choices are Cheerios, Wheat Chex, Wheaties, some Kashi cereals and Farina.

**5)** Bread may be either plain or toasted whole grain, such as whole wheat, whole rye or pumpernickel. If desired, bread may be sprayed with a zero-calorie butter substitute.

**6)** Use only lean cuts of meat trimmed of all visible fat. Poultry should be limited to chicken or turkey breasts (white meat only and skinless). Make sure the turkey bacon you use contains no more than 35 Calories per slice.

**7)** When canned tuna or salmon is specified, use only fish packed in water.

**8)** An unlimited amount of green salad may be eaten, but the salad dressing should be as specified. (Incidentally, in the meal plans Evoo means extra virgin olive oil.)

**9)** Use freely as desired: clear unsweetened coffee, clear unsweetened tea, water, seltzer and any diet soda.

**10)** Use freely as desired: clear soups without fat, bouillon, and seasonings such as mustard, cinnamon, dill, herbs, red and black pepper, curry, vinegar, lemon juice and sections, and dill and sour pickles.

**11)** Any specified snack may be moved to any other part of the day, and/or combined with breakfast, lunch or dinner.

## Keeping It Off

Within five years, more than 90 percent of all dieters regain every pound they have lost.  Why? In most cases it's because after losing weight most people eventually revert to their pre-diet eating and exercising habits, and this inevitably leads to their regaining the weight they lost– and often more. The fact is the less you weigh, the less you need to eat to sustain your lower weight.

A study, published in the Annals of Internal Medicine, that followed 4,000 people for three decades suggests that in the long term, 90 percent of men and 70 percent of women will become overweight.  Interestingly, half of the men and women in the study, who had made it well into adulthood without a weight problem, ultimately also became overweight and a third actually became obese.  The point being that you can never become complacent.  You must continually watch your weight because we are all at risk of becoming overweight.

As mentioned previously, the key to long-term weight control success is knowledge and understanding, combined of course with desire and self-discipline.  I suggest you read ***Weight Maintenance - U.S. Edition*** by Vincent Antonetti, Ph.D. (also published by NoPaperPress) – and absolutely the best weight maintenance book, or eBook, on the market.

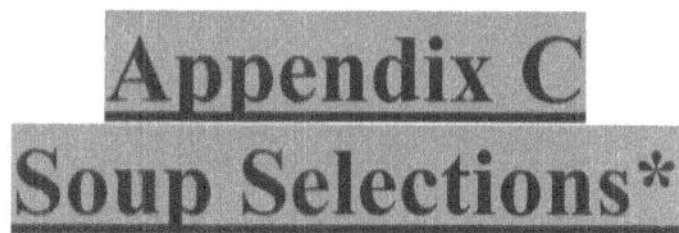

When the Daily Meal Plan menu specifies soup have only one serving (8 ounces) unless stated otherwise.  Note that the listed soup were available in most supermarkets as of 07/24/2020.   *These are a canned soup selections.

| Soup Description | Calories |
| --- | --- |
| Healthy Choice Chicken with Rice | 90 |
| Campbell's Tomato | 100 |
| Healthy Choice Country Vegetable | 100 |
| Progresso Minestrone* | 110 |
| Progresso Chickarina* | 110 |
| Progresso Italian-Style Wedding* | 120 |
| Campbell's Home-Style Light Chicken Corn Chowder* | 120 |
| Campbell's Home-Style Chicken Noodle | 130 |
| Campbell's Home-Style Butter Nut Squash* | 130 |
| Campbell's Healthy Request Vegetable Beef | 140 |
| Progresso Lentil* | 140 |
| Progresso Green Split Pea* | 150 |
| Campbell's Slow Kettle New England Clam Chowder | 160 |
| Progresso Macaroni and Bean* | 160 |
| Progresso New England Clam Chowder* | 170 |
| Progresso Lasagna-Style* | 170 |
| Progresso Broccoli Cheese with Bacon* | 180 |
| Have 2 servings of a 90 Calorie soup | 180 |
| Campbell's Chunky Classic Chicken Noodle | 190 |
| Amy's Rustic Italian Vegetable* | 190 |
| Campbell's Chunky Beef n Cheese* | 200 |
| Amy's French Country Vegetable* | 210 |
| Campbell's Chunky Sirloin Burger + Vegetables | 220 |
| Enjoy two servings of a 110 or 120 Calorie soup | 230 |
| Enjoy two servings of a 120 Calorie soup | 240 |

# <u>NoPaperPress Paperbacks and eBooks</u>

100-Day Super Diet-1200 Calorie*  
100-Day Super Diet-1500 Calorie*  
100-Day No-Cooking Diet-1200 Cal*  
100-Day No-Cooking Diet-1500 Cal*  
90-Day Smart Diet-1200 Calorie*  
90-Day Smart Diet-1500 Calorie*  
90-Day No-Cooking Diet - 1200 Cal*  
90-Day No-Cooking Diet - 1500 Cal*  
90-Day Perfect Diet - 1200 Calorie*  
90-Day Perfect Diet - 1500 Calorie*  
60-Day Perfect Diet-1200 Calorie*  
60-Day Perfect Diet-1500 Calorie*  
50-Day Flex Diet-1200 Calorie*  
50-Day Flex Diet-1500 Calorie*  
30-Day Quick Diet - for Women*  
30-Day Quick Diet - for Men*  
30-Day No-Cooking Diet*  
30-Day Diet for Women - Metric*  
30-Day Diet for Men - Metric*  
25 Day Easy Diet-1200 Calorie*  
25 Day Easy Diet-1500 Calorie*  
25-Day No-Cooking Diet  
10-Day Express Diet  
10-Day No-Cooking Diet*  
7-Day Diet for Women*  
7-Day Diet for Men*  
7-Day No-Cooking Diets*  
90-Day Gluten-Free Diet-1200 Cal*  
90-Day Gluten-Free Diet-1500 Cal*  
30-Day Gluten-Free Quick Diet*  
30-Day Gluten-Free No-Cooking Diet*  
7-Day Diet for Women - Metric*  
7-Day Diet for Men - Metric  
7-Day Gluten-Free Express Diet*  
7-Day Gluten-Free No-Cooking Diet*  
90-Day Vegetarian Diet-1200 Calorie*  
90-Day Vegetarian Diet-1500 Calorie*  
30-Day Vegetarian Diet*  
7-Day Vegetarian Diet*  
Weight Loss for Women*  
Weight Loss for Women - Metric  
Weight Loss for Women - UK  
Weight Loss for Men*  
Maximum Weight Loss - 1200 Cal*  
Maximum Weight Loss - 1500 Cal*  

Weight Loss for Men - Metric*  
Maximum Weight Loss- 1200 Calorie*  
Maximum Weight Loss- 1500 Calorie*  
Weight Control - U.S. Edition  
Weight Control - Metric. Edition  
Professional Weight Control Women - U.S.  
Professional Weight Control Women -  
Professional Weight Control Men - U.S.  
Professional Weight Control Men - Metric  
Weight Maintenance - U.S. Edition*  
Weight Maintenance - Metric. Edition*  
Weight Maintenance - UK Edition  
Weight Loss for Senior Men*  
Weight Loss for Senior Women*  
Eat Smart - U.S. Edition*  
Eat Smart - Metric Edition  
30-Day Mediterranean Diet  
Exercise Smart - U.S. Edition*  
Exercise Smart - Metric Edition  
Exercise Smart - UK Edition*  
Total Fitness - U.S. Edition  
Total Fitness - Metric Edition  
Total Fitness - UK Edition  
Total Fitness for Women-U.S. Edition*  
Total Fitness for Women - Metric  
Total Fitness for Women - UK Edition  
Total Fitness for Men - U.S. Edition*  
Total Fitness for Men- Metric Edition*  
Total Fitness for Men - UK Edition  
Senior Fitness - U.S. Edition*  
Senior Fitness - Metric Edition*  
Senior Fitness - UK Edition*  
Computer Diet - U.S. Edition*  
Computer Diet - Metric Edition*  
Reliable Weight Loss - U.S. Edition  
101 Weight Loss Tips*  
101 Healthy Eating Tips*  
101 Lifelong Fitness Tips*  
101 Weight Maintenance Tips  
101 Weight Loss Recipes  
101 Gluten-Free Weight Loss Recipes  
101 Vegetarian Weight Loss Recipes*  
30-Day Mediterranean Diet*  
90-Day Mediterranean Diet - 1200 Cal*  
90-Day Mediterranean Diet - 1500 Cal*  

* These titles are available as both ebooks and paperbacks. Our ebooks are sold by Amazon, Apple, Google, Barnes & Noble and Kobo. But our paperbacks are only sold by Amazon.

# Disclaimer

This book offers general meal planning, nutrition and weight control information. It is not a medical manual and the author does not claim to be medically qualified. The material in this book is not intended to be a substitute for medical counseling. Everyone should have a medical checkup before beginning a weight loss program. Moreover, the physician conducting the medical exam should be made aware of and should approve the specific weight control program planned. Additionally, while the author and publisher have made every effort to ensure the accuracy of the information in this book, they make no representations or warranties regarding its accuracy or completeness. Further, neither the author nor publisher assume liability for any medical problems that might result from applying the methods in this book, or for any loss of profit, or any other commercial damages, including but not limited to special, incidental, consequential or other damages, and any such liability is hereby expressly disclaimed.